CW01432193

The Holistic Alchemist

Guided Meditations

Anna Everett

Anna Everett - Holistic Alchemist

Anna Everett - Author and Motivational Speaker

www.holisticalchemist.co.uk

www.annaeverettauthor.com

www.maddiemaeauthor.com

Contents

Introduction

Sometimes the idea of meditating is ruined by the inability to find focus, or know what to think to oneself in the quiet moments.

These scripts were all written by me as a resource for my guided meditation classes, however if they are able to help other people find their meditative state then I am more than happy for them to be used at home.

It is up to you if you record them and play them back, or whether you just gain inspiration from reading them. You could sit and read one and then work your way through a meditation based on what you remember.

Please do not get hung up on details, or needed to follow word for word. There is no right and wrong in meditation, it is all about achieving that peace and clarity and allowing your brain to shut off from the hustle and bustle of the daily grind.

On the next page you will find a reminder, taken from my book, The Holistic Alchemist presents.... A Guide to Meditation, just incase you are struggling with setting the scene and getting started.

Meditation is meant to be a happy peaceful time, so remove all stress from yourself. You do not have to sit cross legged, dressed in white, looking like a model for a Zen magazine.

You simply have to be you, and let yourself relax and enjoy what you are doing.

Technically one can meditate anywhere, and I regularly do. I love sitting on a warm beach meditating, a bench by a sunny river, and walking meditation is something I really enjoy, but at home it is great to create a space for yourself to meditate.

As well as giving you somewhere to go - 'right children / partner / pets... I am off to my meditation space now' it also creates an area of purpose. When I am feeling particularly lazy my yoga practice gets pushed to the side of my periphery and it becomes super easy for me to forget and feel no guilt, because as a rule my yoga mat lives under the couch.

However, if I had the luxury of endless space I would create a yoga space and the fact I walk past it to get to other areas of my home would force me to at least feel guilty for not bothering. The same is true of your meditation space. Meditation is often something we mean to do, but somehow forget to do more often than not.

You can of course meditate in bed last thing at night but that will more often than not result in you falling asleep - to a point this is no bad thing but, it shouldn't become the only way you meditate. Creating a space, no matter how small, with a dedicated purpose, makes it more likely that you will remember to complete your meditation.

The area needs to only be a small corner, but needs to be as free from distraction as possible. I have mine set up in a corner of my bedroom, because I find it easiest to meditate when everyone is still awake.

Shutting myself in the bedroom gives me the maximum potential for quiet!

A meditation space should be free from 'blue' light - that is television light, computer monitor, iPad, iPhone - if you are going to use such a device to give you relaxing music - or one of my guided meditations then you should place the device behind you, face down so the screen is not emitting any light.

I like to practice my meditation in natural light or if it has gone dark already soft muted lights from candles or a small lamp.

Blue light is a stimulant to the brain and, being able to see a source of blue light makes it much harder to quiet the mind.

I have on occasion resorted to meditating in the front room amidst the hullabaloo, however this required an eye mask and headphones and really wasn't ideal.

Your meditation space should be a reflection of you, and your desire to learn about your mind. My Buddhist leanings see my corner made up of Tibetan Prayer Flags, a statue of Buddha and some candles. A simple cushion on the floor is enough to sit on or for those with reduce mobility, whatever chair makes you feel comfortable and rested. My corner is near my bed, and I will often sit on the bed, but I take care not to lay down, (suggesting to my brain that it is time to sleep!)

There is no right or wrong way to sit for meditation. You can lay down, but as I say, I find this too close to sleep positioning and then often drop off before I can complete my meditation. Traditionally you will see meditating people depicted cross legged, or on short stools, known as meditation stools which look slightly uncomfortable. Again this was a bit of a cunning plan to ensure they remained aware throughout and didn't get so comfortable they nodded off.

It is perfectly acceptable to sit on a chair, or sit with your legs out. The golden rule is simply don't cross the legs (unless you sit in Lotus a lot) else you will end up with pins and needles that will quite cheerfully ruin your session!

Depending on your heating you may find, sat still for a period, you feel chilly. Lots of people keep a jumper or blanket in the meditation corner and pop that on before they begin. I love my blankets and drape one around my shoulders before I begin.

Your meditation space should be for you alone, and for the soul purpose of meditation, so if you have a table there with your pretty things one, resist the temptation to plonk down a coffee mug, or some post, it needs to remain clear.

An excellent idea I stumbled upon a few years back, for those who are really short of space, or those who have inquisitive toddlers that just can't resist touching, is a meditation tray. A decorative tray with a lip / sides to prevent things sliding. You can set up your pretty things there - your candles, statues etc, and then simply lift clear out of harms way and store on top of a cupboard until needed.

If at all possible it is great if you can have the space in an open area where lots of air can circulate. In the summer I have the bedroom windows open, I can smell nature which makes a deeper connection to the earth.

It is also important to be able to clean the space of stale air and stagnant energy between uses. So, even if it would be too cold to meditate with windows open, ensure you allow air in there at other times to clear your space and keep it healthy.

I like to create a nice scented area so will often burn a scented candle or incense stick whilst I meditate, you can use a specific scent to work with your meditation or if you have nothing to link into the meditation just something you really like the aroma of!

So now you are almost ready to begin - exciting isn't it :) - if you can possibly cope without it, leave you mobile somewhere else in the house, at very least have it on silent.

The first thing we need to do before we meditate is ground ourselves.

Grounding is a tool that connects you to the earth, the ground where we all come from and must one day return, and allows you to connect to the earths energy rather than deplete your own. Now, I realise to some of you this sounds like a very strange premise, however, it is common practice, and if you like good practice in meditation.

It takes just a couple of minutes, and I ground myself before I do anything else.

Make yourself comfortable, in the position you have chosen to meditate. Close your eyes and imagine yourself standing on the earth. Bare earth, bare feet. Your actual location or position of your feet is irrelevant, you are using visualisation. As you stand both feet firmly on the bare earth, imagine roots coming from your feet and heading down into the earth below. See them taking root and pushing deeper into the ground below.

At the end of the session you can see the roots returning to your body, leaving the earth. Remember to thank the earth for its energy and allowing you to be part of it. As trivial as this sounds it does work, give it a try and see for yourself.

Breathing

Before you begin a meditation you can first start by focusing your attention on your breathing. Yoga, which has close links to meditation, offers a number of breathing exercises. Both used in yoga and meditation class, these exercises will help you relax and calm your breathing and begin to create a state of single focus, so vital in meditation.

As I already mentioned in relation to breathing meditations, our normal status quo breathing is pretty poor. When you first start to practice breathing exercising you need to use short sessions, as you may find you become slightly light headed and dizzy. Our lungs have the capacity to hold significantly more air than we give them credit for. If I asked you to get on a treadmill and run, until you could run no more...(I wont don't worry!) there would come a point where your lungs actually started working at full capacity.

Now clearly we don't want to spend our whole lives in a breathless state of running just to use our lungs properly. It is actually perfectly possible to learn to use our lungs properly from a state total relaxation and bliss.

As you practice these breathing exercises keep in mind the light headed stuff - always rest a few moments after to allow your breathing to return to normal before getting up. Those with high blood pressure should not hold their breath.

4-7-8 Breathing exercise

Alternate nostril breathing

Belly breathing

4-7-8 is a very well known breathing exercise, it is sometimes called relaxation breath.

You can practice this sitting or laying, and it is said to be excellent for panic attack sufferers, so, if this is you, try and teach this to your partner and close friends and ask them to try and coach you through this should a panic attack strike. (Panic attacks are horrible, cloud the brain and leave you unable to function. I have first hand experience and will discuss panic attacks and anxiety more in my book 'The Holistic Alchemist presents Calm and relaxed') Teach this breathing exercise to your nearest and dearest and remind them you will NOT be cooperative and they will have to work hard to get you to comply!

But, in a relaxed calm state of mind you can practice this breathing on your own, it is nice and simple, and the numbers give us a clue as to what we are going to do!

Breathe in through your nose for a count of 4

Hold your breath for a count of 7

Breathe out through your mouth for a count of 8

Repeat 4 times.

As you inhale through the nose your breath is silent. As you exhale through the mouth you create a purposeful audible release of air.

Alternate Nostril Breathing

This is a classic and favourite yogic breathing exercise of mine. Again this can be done sitting or laying down. I prefer to be seated.

This one is a bit more complicated but here goes!

Use your right thumb and middle finger.

Block your right nostril with your thumb

Inhale for a count of 4

Block your left nostril and hold your breath for a count of 4

Release your right thumb and exhale through your right nostril for a count of 4

Leave your left nostril blocked and inhale through your right nostril for a count of 4

Block your right nostril with your thumb again and hold your breath for a count of 4

Release your left nostril and exhale for a count of 4

So, your breath is only flowing through one nostril at a time, and alternating. Inhale left, exhale right, inhale right, exhale left.

Again perform the circuit 4 times and then return to normal breathing. This is also useful for panic attacks, or for general relaxation.

Belly breathing

I personally prefer to practice belly breathing laying down, as it is easier to monitor what I am doing.

This exercise I find really highlights just how poor my breathing becomes when I go about my daily life. If I skip this exercise for a few days it is so much harder to do when I return to it.

This exercise is best practiced laying on your back. Start by putting one hand on your belly, and the other hand on your chest. Now exhale through your open mouth to empty your lungs. Pause, and inhale deeply through your mouth. As you inhale you need to aim to inflate your stomach as if it were a balloon. Your hands resting on your body will show you how well your stomach is rising. Pause again and exhale through the mouth allowing the stomach to deflate and return to normal. Repeat about 4 times, seeing how big you can get your stomach! Once you finish the exercise allow your breathing to return to normal, and if you are getting up, do so slowly.

You can use the breathing exercises as a pre-meditation warm up, and if you are ready you can begin your meditation from here. If you still feel chaotic and flustered then continue on with the relaxation exercise.

The relaxation exercise will be done laying down, on your back. Get yourself comfortable, and make sure you will not be cold, use a blanket if required. Now begin at your toes. Really clench the muscles, curl the toes forward, create as much tension as possible, then release. We are going to continue in this manner focusing our attention up through the body.

Now focus on the legs, tense your leg muscles, so you feel your kneecaps pull up towards your torso. Squeeze the muscles as tight as possible and release. Now your glut muscles, the muscles of the bum, squeeze them as tight as you can and release. Turn your focus to your stomach area, pull in your stomach as much as you can, hold it as tight as possible and then release. Now your shoulders and chest, tighten the muscles, create tension and release. Move now to the arms. Ball your fingers into a fist, tuck your elbows into your body, create the tension, and release.

Finally the head and face, screw up your eyes so they are tightly shut, force a big fake grin, feel the tension and release.

Now picture yourself laying on the softest of mattresses and try and imagine your body sinking into the mattress as it takes the weight and supports all of you, a weightless feeling free from tension. Lay for a few minutes enjoying the relaxation.

You are now ready to meditate. You can either remain laying down or return yourself to a seated position but if possible go straight in to the mediation from here as you have already begun to relax the body. This exercise can also be used at night before you sleep to rid the body of the stress of the day, when you finish simply turn to your normal sleeping position and drift off.

In order to achieve the best effects please ensure you have created a quiet space where you are not likely to be interrupted. As with all meditative experiences, should you need to return to full awareness to attend to any matter you will be able to do so instantly and safely.

Please do not attempt to use this track whilst driving or operating machinery.

This meditation can be enjoyed in a seated position or laying down, which ever is most comfortable.

Please do not cross your arms or legs.

We are now ready to begin.

Anxiety

In order to get the maximum benefit from the meditation you first need to
create yourself a totally relaxed state, clearing your mind of the hustle
and bustle of daily life. Once you find a comfortable place, simply close
your eyes and concentrate on calming your breathing. We all normally
breathe at a rate that is faster than we should breathe, this is because
most of the time we are not focusing on it at all.

Lets move our breathing into the spotlight by focusing on a count of 4.
Inhale for a count of 4.....1....2.....3....4......and exhale for a count of
4......1....2.....3......4.... Inhale for a count of 4.....1....2.....3....4......
and exhale for a count of 4......1.....2.....3......4......every time you
exhale try and release all tension and stress from the body, Inhale for a
count of 4.....1....2.....3....4......and exhale for a count of 4......1.....
2.....3......4.... tensions escaping now, you are slowly feeling calmer
and more relaxed.

Concentrate on your breathing and nothing else, empty your mind of all
other thoughts as these can wait, instead we will use meditation and the
magical power of imagination to take a journey to new wonderful places
where stress doesn't exist and where you can concentrate the mind and
really enjoy being in a meditative state.

Now as you look around in your minds eye, you find yourself in a white room. A warm and inviting soft white sofa appears in front of you, and you stroll slowly over and sit down. Still taking in the sights around you.

On one wall is a beautiful ornate fireplace, with logs cracking and popping gently as they burn. The orange of the fire is the only colour in the room.

The room is deeply relaxing and peaceful.

Slowly a screen is lowered down in front of you, a large white television screen on a large white arm.

As the screen flickers to life you see yourself on the screen. The thing about this you, is that you have no anxieties and fears. You can see yourself in your favourite place, smiling, happy - you are positively glowing with happiness. All your negativities simply don't exist here, you are a whirlwind of positive energy, you are free from worry, and you look awesome.

You sit and watch the screen, totally glued to the images in front of you, look at yourself, it really is you but you look so much happier. Your face looks younger, this is because anxiety ages us, but you are glowing, radiant and youthful.

Look at what you are wearing, even your clothes look brighter, freeing yourself from anxiety has clearly had a knock on effect to other areas of your life, it is as though you are taking so much more care with your appearance. No tired faded, threadbare clothes in sight, this version of you has clearly taken time and effort to select the clothes and this version of you looks totally amazing.

You are groomed and fresh. Look at how your smile really is so totally radiant. The transformation in your appearance is completely remarkable. It slowly dawns on you that this is your future, this is totally achievable, you thought it wasn't, but here in front of you is the proof that is really is possible. As you watch yourself doing the things you love surrounded by your friends and family, you smile at the screen.

This version of you on the screen, this radiant person, this anxiety free version of you is smiling too, they are so happy and full of positive energy. Notice how you look so relaxed, even your posture has changed. You head is held hight, and your shoulders are back, you are a perfect picture of confidence and happiness. This version of you is making eye contact with those around you, no longer hiding, lost in your own anxious thoughts. Now notice how the people you are with are treating you.

Everyone wants to be in your presence, they have recognised the difference in you and they like it. Everyone around you is pleased for you, it brings joy to your loved ones to see you free from stress, they felt sad and worried at your suffering when you were at your most anxious. Now they are delighted to see the change in you and enjoy sharing it with you as you enjoy this life, free from anxiety and fear.

You completely love watching the images as they play out in front of you. The scenes start to change, and as you watch, you now see yourself living and loving your life. As this transformed version of you goes about their day see how in control of this life they are. No longer are you fearful or worried about anything. This you is peaceful and relaxed in every situation. Simply letting stress slide off you like water off a duck's back.

Anxiety is not created anymore because you now know how to deal with it and make it stop before it has a chance to take hold. You calmly stroll away from any situation that has the potential to distress you or cause stress to rise. Instead you choose no to concentrate on the things in your life that make you feel happy. You are a good seeking missile of positivity. Negativity has no place in your life anymore and you find it easy, so very easy to let go of worries and cares, simply let them float away.

You do not need anxiety so you do not accept anxiety. You are having such a great time watching yourself on the television screen, it is so wonderful to see yourself brimming with optimism and strength, facing the world with such a great attitude towards everything and everyone you come into contact with. You marvel at this version of you on the screen before you. This transformed you is just amazing and you handle every situation with ease and confidence. This person is exactly who you want to be and what is even better is the knowledge that this really is you.

You are going to grow into this version of you, and that is a really exciting thought. You lean forwards nearer to the screen wanting to absorb every moment, as you do so a white light surrounds you and you are picked up and taken into the screen itself, floating into the scene you saw before, into your new anxiety free body. You are now there, part of this amazing life, your life, this really is fantastic.

You notice immediately how brilliant you feel, knowing that you have conquered the stress and it is gone forever. You feel calmer and much more in control. It is an awesome state. As you move around talking to friends and family you feel so happy and confident. Your old anxieties and worries seem to be a life time away, there is nothing here but happiness.

Gone is the fear, gone is the stress, replaced with this new inner peace that leaves you happy and relaxed. You look through your eyes as if they were new eyes, yes, yes this is how you are going to be from now on. You know without a doubt that you can achieve this transformation and really become this version of you. You tell yourself how much you love these new feelings of positivity and that you are going to bring them back to the present day with you. This, you say to yourself, this is my new life, and it starts now.

You close your eyes for the briefest of moments and find yourself sat back on the white sofa, feeling so peaceful and so positive with a new determination to succeed.

It is now time to leave this place, time to return the mind to the present day once more, time to return to your body as you rest in meditation.

The room fades and you feel yourself returning to the present moment, once more return your concentrate to your breathing. Inhale for a count of 4.....1....2.....3....4......and exhale for a count of 4......1.....2.....

3......4.... Inhale for a count of 4.....1....2.....3....4......and exhale for a count of 4......1.....2.....3......4......

You will feel like you have just awoken from a deep refreshing sleep, you will feel rested and revived and totally at peace with yourself. Stretching out the body now, just as you have seen a cat do when awakening from a nap, stretch every muscle, every limb, feeling so good now.

You can return to your day aware that you have made the first step to a less anxious you and learnt a new meditation trick to help your keeping building on this new found learning until you have successfully eliminated all the anxieties from your life.

Building Self Confidence

In order truly enjoy and get the best from any meditation you first need to create a completely peaceful state and clear your mind of the hustle and bustle of daily life. Once you have found your comfortable place, close your eyes and focus on calming your breathing. Normal respiration is often much faster than we should breathe, however we rarely take time to focus on it.

Try and slow your breathing by focusing on the count of 4. Inhale for a count of 4.....1....2.....3....4......and exhale for a count of 4......1..... 2.....3......4.... Inhale for a count of 4.....1....2.....3....4......and exhale for a count of 4......1.....2.....3......4......every time you exhale try and release all tension and stress from the body, Inhale for a count of 4..... 1....2.....3....4......and exhale for a count of 4......1.....2.....3......4.... tensions escaping now, feeling calmer and more relaxed.

Just concentrate on your breathing, emptying your mind of all those thoughts that can easily wait and use the meditation and use the power of your imagination to take you to brilliant places.

Wonderful places where stress doesn't exist and where you can develop your mind and being in the safety of a meditative state.

Now I want you to concentrate your mind on the idea of a beautiful walled garden, you have entered the garden from a small archway on one side, and you stroll in under the arch and stand and look around. You feel instantly completely at ease here, you cannot believe how peaceful it feels just by entering this fantastic space, right in the middle of the garden is a bench and I would like you now to stroll over and sit on the bench.

The lush green grass feels amazingly soft beneath your bare feet as you wander lazily across the lawns to reach the beach. You reach the beach and sit yourself down, making yourself comfortable. You can now have a proper look around this garden. It is a lovely warm summer day, the sun is shining brightly and warming your head and shoulders. You can hear the gentle sound of bird song as they too enjoy this wonderful place.

As you look around you can see that the garden is completely walled on all sides, a locked solid gate in one corner, and the arch way you came through being the only other entrance to the garden. It is a completely private space, and you are alone here, and happy in your own company, it is a place of complete tranquility.

The lush green grass, the flowers and shrubs, the birds singing, it really is a beautiful place, how can you feel anything but happy here.

You become aware of the sound of gently trickling water, looking around you locate an ornamental fountain splashing into a small pool. In the pond a few large goldfish swim lazily around, almost as of they too are effected by the wonderful relaxation this garden creates, it is sublimely hypnotic and you feel quite sleepy just sat there enjoying the surroundings.

Perhaps you will just sit here all day enjoying the peace and beauty of the garden. You are enjoying the feeling of being totally relaxed, listening to the birds singing, the fountain splashing and watching the gentlest of breezes moving the trees and flowers.

Sat here it is easy to feel confident about yourself, so now we will learn a meditation trick that helps us to transfer that feeling back to daily life, and help you have a positive self image. It is something you can practice often until being self confident and not worrying about the opinions of others becomes second nature. It is a powerful and clever trick that you can take back into your daily life.

There is so much media information about the perfect body, the perfect look, the perfect job, the perfect relationship, it is all too easy for us to get caught up with comparing ourselves to the media images, and feeling jealous of the lives of others. At work, in daily life, other people seem so together and confident they just seem to shine and it makes you feel inferior and somehow not as good.

It is now time to banish those thoughts from the mind forever, they are not real, they are simply things we have created by worrying and comparing ourselves to others. It makes no difference if you are hung up on your physical image, your personality, your ability to succeed at work, now it really is time to stop and learn how to love yourself once more. You are an fantastic unique person - there is only one if you in this world, you really are truly unique and that is an fantastic thing.

As you sit in the beautiful garden a mirror appears in front of you. When you look in the mirror at first you see only yourself as a child. This is because when you were a very young child you were free of the trappings of life. Self image and belief in oneself are not things that even come into being a child. See the young child in front of you reflected in the mirror, carefree and happy, smiling and dancing. A toddler never worries about their weight, their looks, their confidence.

When a toddler sees themselves in a mirror they simply smile and play with the image. The toddler in you is smiling. Looking at this carefree child makes you smile, that is good, smile at the toddler as they play so carefree and unaffected by the world. As you continue to look into the mirror, the image of the toddler fades and you can now see yourself as you are today. Keep smiling, there is no reason to stop. The version of you, you see is still you, and you are beautiful and unique.

Remember the toddler, the toddler in you is smiling. Believe that you have a right to smile now too. Looking at yourself as you are now makes you smile, you are special and unique no matter what you might once have thought. You can learn to like and believe in yourself once more just as you did when you were a child.

Every time a negative thought or image creeps into view in the mirror immediately call back the toddler and watch them playing once more.

Listen to the birds over head, remember how at peace you feel in this garden. Dealing with your own confidence can be hard work but you can conquer this as you grow a belief in your ability and strength.

Look into the mirror again now as see you as you are today, smile at yourself, be kind to yourself, repeat to yourself 'I love and approve of myself, I am confident and believe in myself'.

It is much more common than you might think to struggle with ones self confidence, you are certainly not alone and you should never feel bad that you are find this difficult.

For a moment I want you to refocus your attention on the garden, the beautiful garden, notice again the warmth of the sun, remember how peaceful and relaxed you feel here. It is easier to feel confident when you are feeling calm, now you are feeling really peaceful again we will take this feeling back with us as we look in the mirror once more.

There you are, looking at your reflection and smiling because you are amazing, repeat to yourself 'I love and approve of myself, I am confident and believe in myself'. If any negative thoughts or feelings begin to creep in, summon that inner child, revel in the innocence, laugh with them as they play, as they clap and smile, giggling at the reflection in the mirror - look how much they love you.

You can love you too, simply because you are a wonderful and unique person. See how much easier this becomes the more you do it, the more you look at yourself through the eyes of a child and the more you smile and laugh with your inner child. You are an amazing person. You are truly unique and that is a great thing. repeat to yourself 'I love and approve of myself, I am confident and believe in myself'

The final step on your journey is to see one more reflection in that mirror, the reflection of the ideal confident you that you want to become.

Focus on creating that version of you. What do you want to see, what do you want to be. Have you changed your appearance? Is you hair different? Are you clothes different? Is this about your physical appearance or how you interact with other people, your mind and how your choose to think?

Whatever it is you want to change, see yourself, with those changes now made reflected in the mirror, smile at that person, say hello to that version of you, that is you. The you that you are going to become very soon, are already becoming, the confident you that does not struggle with their physical appearance or their ability to deal with other people. Look at that you and smile repeat to yourself 'I love and approve of myself, I am confident and believe in myself'.

Look how even more amazing you are when you have self confidence, you can be that version of yourself, you will be that version of you. It is within your control and something you can achieve by embracing the inner child and learning from them, letting them teach you to love yourself again, just as you did before life battered and bruised you, before the trappings of life jaded you and brought about doubt.

Look around you again, you are still in the warmth and safety of the garden, you can still hear birds singing and the fountain bubbling. You can return to this place whenever you wish by summoning the child within you, and when you think about that child, no matter where you are or what you are doing, you will also be able to hear the sounds of the garden and feel the warmth, this will create the safe relaxed state that you have right now, and this state of mind is perfect for learning and shaping ourselves and developing this new self confident you.

You have begun an important journey and by coming back and repeating this meditation you will soon reach your journeys end and will struggle to remember a time when you were not as confident as you have become. You will be transported back to this fantastic place every time you say to yourself 'I love and approve of myself, I am confident and believe in myself' This is your safe place and should a situation ever become uncomfortable and you find your confidence waining you can always use this trick to return here to recharge yourself, even for the briefest of moments.

Even in a crowded room surrounded by people, you can return here momentarily to find that peaceful feeling you need to summon the more confident you.

For now, sadly our experience in the garden must come to an end, however you can take this feeling of deep contentment and peaceful with you when you return to your day and your busy life once more. Simply keep remembering the garden and your bench. For now you must leave your bench, crossing the garden back to the archway. Feeling the soft grass beneath your feet as you walk to the archway. The sounds of the fountain fading as you leave them behind.

It is time to return your mind to your present once more, to your body as you relax in meditation. Feel yourself returning to the present moment and once more focus on your breathing. Inhale for a count of 4.....1.... 2.....3....4......and exhale for a count of 4......1.....2.....3......4.... Inhale for a count of 4.....1....2.....3....4......and exhale for a count of 4...... 1.....2.....3......4...... You will feel like you have just awoken from a deep refreshing slumber, you will feel rested and revived and totally at peace with yourself.

Stretching out your body now, just as you have seen a cat awakening from a nap, stretch every muscle, every limb, feeling so good now. You can return to your day aware that you have made the first step to a more self confident you and learnt a new meditation trick to help your keeping building on this new found learning until you have created the perfect self confident you.

Dealing with stress

To begin I would like you to close your eyes and just concentrate on relaxing every muscle in your body. Beginning with your feet imagine you are becoming heavier and heavier, a nice warm relaxing heavy. Feel your feet sinking into the ground or into bed beneath you.

Now concentrate your attention on your ankles, feel the warmth spreading and radiating up to your lower legs, up to your knees and radiating up to the thighs. This is the laziest heavy state you can ever remember, and you are not required to do anything but relax and enjoy this experience.

The warm relaxing feeling now spreading up through your hips, pelvis and buttocks. Radiating into your stomach and torso. You start to feel the tensions and stresses of the day just fading away as the relaxation continues up through your body, into the chest and shoulders.

Enjoy how you are feeling as the wave of warmth and heaviness continues to the neck and head, we do not allow ourselves enough time in the daily race to just be at one with ourselves, so cherish this time.

The sense of heavy relaxation continues down your shoulders to the arms, elbows, wrists and fingers.

Now turn your attention to your breathing. I want you to imagine a candle flame flickering just in front of you. As you breathe in, the candle flame remains motionless, as you exhale it dances around.

Control your breath so the candle remains still for a count of four and dances for a count of four, inhale 1, 2, 3, 4 now exhale 1, 2, 3, 4. again, inhale 1, 2, 3, 4 now exhale 1, 2, 3, 4. As you bring your breathing under control more of the stresses of daily life will ebb away leaving you completely at peace. Just breathing in and out, in and out, watching the candle flame dance and flicker.

Now you have created such a relaxed state it is time to begin your meditation. Time to enjoy this state and learn about how it can help you as you go about your daily life. Now just clear your mind of all thoughts, think about nothing but the candle flame flickering back and forth, back and forth. If any unwanted thoughts start to creep in simply turn them away and refocus on the candle. There is plenty of time to deal with any other thoughts and issues later.

Now your mind is clear, and your body and mind are calm, this is the perfect mental state from which to address any difficulties you may discover along the journey of life.

Remember these feelings, remember being so relaxed, so devoid of stress and tension, add this to your memory bank, this feeling of complete and utter relaxation and contentment.

Should the need arise you can recreate this feeling at anytime by simply remembering that candle flame flickering gently back and forth, back and forth. This is a skill you can practice anytime, anywhere, wherever stress and tension may arise. Just clear your mind and focus on that candle flame, people around you may even start to comment how peaceful and chilled out your are.

The candle flame focus allows you time to process the situation without getting caught up in any stresses and tensions that have arisen. Focus intently on that candle now, remember how it moves, how it looks, how it smells, these are the cues that you can use to bring yourself back to this state whenever the need arises.

This is part of the art of feeling peaceful and relaxed when stressful emotions arise and by practising this technique both here and now with this meditation and in daily life whenever you can spare the time, you are creating a strong framework for yourself, learning new ways of dealing with stressful situations.

Sadly we will find ourselves experiencing all kinds of stress at various points during our lives, and this is just part of living. By using these powerful meditation techniques you will soon be able to bring about feelings of peace and peaceful no matter what situation arises. In your current state it is hard to imagine how stressed you can become,you are so relaxed and calm, but I want you now to imagine a situation that causes a minor amount of stress, nothing serious just a small annoyance that might cause you minor stress.

Now in your peaceful and calm state of being I want you to encapsulate that stress into a golden ball of light. Just wrapped up in light to form a golden orb, concentrate on the golden light until it has completely surround the problem or situation that causes you stress. The golden ball of light serves two purposes, not only does it hold that stressful situation away from you, allowing you some distance and clarity of thought, but it helps transforms any negative emotions into positive powerful emotions that can be used to create your calmness in crisis.

37

By practicing this technique now you will be better prepared to face the challenges of any new stressful situations that arise. It does not matter where your stress arises, this new trick can assist you in managing any stress in any environment, be that at work, at home, on the road, wherever you may be, the uses of this golden light are endless.

Any situation you are not happy with can be treated in this way. Now for just a moment lets return to that situation once more, your minor stress situation. It remains where you left it, you encapsulated that situation in a golden ball of light. Using the power of your mind you can now shrink that ball of light so it is no bigger than a football.

You can now easily hold that golden ball of light in your hands, reach forward and do that now, your stressful situation has become as small as a football, isn't that amazing it is no longer massive and overpowering. Hold it now, you are now empowered - how brilliant is this, you are doing amazingly well.

This situation and all of the emotions associated with it are now firmly within your control. This situation that once left you stressed, maybe anxious and distressed is now yours to control, yours to take responsibility over and the best bit is you can.

Holding onto your ball of golden light, you can now look into the situation with outside eyes, detached and uninvolved. Look how small and insignificant you have made it look closely, you have done that.

Pause again a moment to enjoy and revel in your peaceful and relaxed state, your candle flame is still there flickering away. Enjoy that state, you feel warm and peaceful and happy.

Now return your concentration and energy to that ball of light. Using your outside eyes you can wander around the situation from a position of complete calm. Look calmly at your situation you have wrapped in golden light. It seems so small and insignificant now. Look for the good and the positive. Consider this now tiny situation before you and know that there is a way to handle the stress and negativity. You have taken control and responsibility for your feelings.

You do not have to let this situation upset you because you have full control over how you react. You can learn new ways of reacting, you can send old panicky stressful responses away for ever and create new patterns of behaviour that you do want. That is not to say situations will not arise that are distressing however your reaction is what defines how much stress you suffer.

A situation cannot carry a certain amount of stress, a situation can only be as stressful as the amount of tension and stress you place on it. You used to empower the stress, now you are going to remove all power and only empower yourself and the way you deal with a situation. Focus on the candle flame and remember you have complete control

You are in control of your reactions to any given situations.

Breathe in for a count of 4, and exhale for a count of 4. Watch the flame flicker and you exhale and repeat internally 'I am in control of my reactions to any situation' 'I am in control of my reactions to any situation'.

Now return your focus to the ball of golden light once more. You are now able to choose how you will react to your situation, you have the power and strength to shrink this stress and make it manageable. Your last step on your journey of control is to now throw the ball of golden light as high as you can up in to the air above you.

Throw that ball now, throw it high. Watching it soar up above your head and then instead of simply falling, just as it reaches its highest point, it explodes like a beautiful firework. Shards of pretty golden light fall in all directions, dispelling and stress and negativity you feel about this situation and sending little diamonds of positive energy back down to surround you.

Now you can sit back and watch this wonderful display of light you have created, watch the fireworks display as it dispels your stressful situation to the four corners of the earth. Bask in the golden light and in these amazing feelings of relaxation and control you have created.

Relaxed and controlled is a powerful combination and you are now a force to be reckoned with when it comes to stressful situations. You can practice these techniques at any time, you can replay this meditation at any time. The more you practise the stronger you will be and the easier it will seem to take control of a stressful situation as it arises.

Congratulate yourself on your ability to learn a new skill, never underestimate the importance of acknowledging your own achievement even if they seem quite small and insignificant. You have done fantastic things here today and taken great steps to regain control and responsibility for your reactions in stressful situations. Well done. Now you can take a brief moment to enjoy the candle flame before it is time to leave this place.

Gaze at that candle flame, it is so pretty and bright, and something so pretty and bright must surely be a positive trick. A positive trick you have created and can summon at any time to help you whenever the need arises. Your beautiful candle flame that remains firmly attached to the feelings of deep calm and relaxation and evert time you visualise your candle those feelings will at once return.

Now it is time to leave this place. Slowly and gently we reverse the process we started with.

Beginning at your toes once more it is time to wake up slowly and gently, start by moving your feet, you can feel them becoming lighter once more, moving up the legs and knees, hips and thighs, you feel refreshed and content. Moving on up through the torso and chest all feelings of heaviness fading being replaced by a warm sense of light and joy. Moving down from the shoulders into the arms and elbows, wrists and fingers. Wiggle your fingers and notice how light they feel now.

Finally return your focus to your head and neck. It is time to wake up now and you can do this with ease. Your whole body feeling light and bright, happy and refreshed. Returning to full awareness once more, eye open and ready to face the day. Enjoy!

Sleep 1

Close your eyes and allow the room to fade as you become alone with your thoughts. The first thing you need to do is relax your body. Allow the tensions of the day to fade and just concentrate on releasing tension from every part of your body.

Imagine yourself at the top of a flight of five stairs and, at the bottom of those stairs is the largest, softest, most inviting feather bed you have ever seen. Look how comfortable it looks and by walking down those five steps you can have the bed all to yourself for complete relaxation.

Step down the first step and as you do so let more tension leave your body, step two, leave all thoughts of your day behind they can wait, right now you and your relaxation are all that matter.

Step three, relaxation is building, feeling tired but happy, a warm and comfortable tired. Step four, you are feeling so relaxed and calm, you just want to lay in the bed and relax now. Step five, the bed is in front of you, lay down now and just feel the luxury of every part of your body sinking into the soft feather down.

The bed creates a comfortable support around you holding you. You are becoming so relaxed and negativity free it is a lovely state, one you want to hold onto and relish.

It is so nice to escape from the day and just take some time to nourish and look after yourself, enjoy this state. Shift your weight gently and notice how the feathers move with you keeping you cushioned and cocooned in their safety and warmth.

It is a lovely warmth that only serves to relax you further. All too often we deny ourselves the chance to relax and do nothing, we feel compelled to keep working away, meeting the impossible demands we place on ourselves. This is why meditation is so important as we need to take the time to look after ourselves, forgetting to take time out is one of the biggest reasons we stop sleeping properly and wake unrefreshed and tired.

In order to sleep properly we must first learn how to clear our mind daily and allow ourselves the opportunity to sleep well. In this wonderfully relaxed state of being it is now time for you to learn some meditation techniques to help you rest better and awaken more refreshed.

Using this meditation you will be able to reach new levels of rest and relaxation. It is now time to begin, and what better way to begin that to create your very own tranquil place of rest. You have already found this fantastic feather bed to hold you and support you, now in your minds eye look around this wonderful room you now find yourself in.

The room is decadent and tranquil, you feel totally safe here. On the opposite side of the room to the bed is a lovely fireplace, the flames dancing mesmerically and the logs popping and crackling as they create the heat to keep you warm. The large heavy deep green velvet curtains are closed over the window to shut out the dark of the night sky, the room has a brilliant feeling that leaves you feeling peaceful and relaxed, peaceful and at ease with yourself. See yourself in this wonderful room, be there now and enjoy the deep sense of relaxation it creates.

It is now time to clear the mind and mentally switch off, for only by doing this can you really have a restful night of deep replenishing sleep. You are now going to learn a mental exercise to help you do just that. I want you to think of a child, who has been playing with toys, the toys are all scattered around the room, but bedtime has arrived.

The scene is chaotic, just like our thoughts can become when we try and rest at night. Like toys from the box they spill out all over creating untidy chaos, is it any surprise then when we cannot sleep? Before the child is taken to bed he is encouraged to tidy the toys back into the box, and that is what I want you to do now with your thoughts.

In your minds eye picture a wooden chest, with a heavy lid, currently it sits open and empty.

You do not need to leave your warm and comfy feather bed, you can do this with the power of your mind. Gather all your thoughts from the day and begin to move them one by one into the chest. Worries about work, worries about money, all go into the chest. worries about family, worries about health, all go into the chest, worries about worries about nothing and everything, all go into the chest.

Clear the thoughts and the chaos is removed, your mind can return to a clear peaceful state, a much better state for achieving the healing rest your body needs and wants. Clear up those thoughts and dump them all into the chest. There is nothing you can do to solve them overnight, but your rest is so important for your mind and your physical health.

Feeling fully rested and revived every morning will be a much greater strength to you than feeling drained and tired. For this moment and for the rest of the night you are going to be only in the present. Today is over, the past cannot be changed and tomorrow can wait. Only the present moment is important.

As you snuggle down into that feather bed you can feel the wonderful sleepy feeling just before sleep, it is getting stronger with every thought and worry you put away into the toy chest.

You need to move every thought, every extraneous thought that creeps into your mind into the chest. Move them over and enjoy the sleepy state that comes from having a clear mind. When all the thoughts have been moved to the chest, close the lid. The box cannot be opened again until the morning. Enjoy the state of an empty mind as you snuggling in that feather bed.

Now you have emptied your mind you can create your sleep barrier. In your mind imagine you are protecting that empty thought space by creating a barrier right round it. Any thoughts that begin to creep in will hit that barrier and be unable to trouble you. No worries at all should enter your being. Now your mind is empty sleep will come.

Do not worry about what the time is, do not work out how long it will be before the alarm goes off, these are thoughts that we cannot allow past the barrier so simply push them back. Remember that all thoughts need to be shut into the toy box. If they will not allow you to push them back then you need to go back through the process again. Open the lid and dump these persistent thoughts back in. You do not need them.

Remember today is over, the past cannot be changed and tomorrow can wait. Only the present moment is important.

You have plenty of time to sleep, and you will now be able to do so with ease as you have cleared your being and emptied the space that previously stopped you from getting the quality of rest you needed. That can now become a thing of the past, you now have a trick to help you clear you mind, a trick that will become stronger the more you practice using it, and you can do this from the safe comfort of your deep feather bed. You can teach yourself how to empty your mind using the toy chest in the corner of the room. All from the safety of your feather bed.

Peaceful and relaxed, happy and sleepy, all your rogue thoughts can be shut safely away each night, simply remembering that today is over, the past cannot be changed and tomorrow can wait, only the present moment is important. This process needs to be practised until it becomes an automatic thing that happens before you shut your eyes at night.

With this trick there will be no fear of how long you have left to sleep, no clock watching, no checking just resting. You will be able to rest peacefully and refreshingly each night waking beautifully refreshed each morning.

Now you know this clever meditation technique you will be able to have such a higher quality of sleep, you will be able to see so clearly that worrying is nothing more than a waste of time as it solves nothing but creates the disturbed sleep that is so detrimental to you, you deserve a brilliant night of rest every night, and you are going to learn how to bring that to yourself by practising this technique over and over until it becomes and automatic process that you don't even have to think about.

And then once your mind has become a clear space you will find sleep comes naturally and easily. In fact some nights you will not even remember the moment you dropped off as you will have created such a peaceful and relaxed state it will just happen before you even know.

You will awaken in this morning feeling refreshed and happy.

It is now time to leave our meditative state and return to the day, which will be just as we left it, you see worrying really does not make a difference or change anything.

Only the present moment is important, the past cannot be changed and tomorrow can wait.

Now you need to begin to get ready to leave your room but remember this is your safe space and you can return here each night, back to your warming fire, back to your heavy velvet curtains and the safety and support of that feather bed that cradles you and keeps you secure and cosy. Time now to stretch and enjoy the feeling of warmth that can only be achieved through full relaxation.

As you begin stretching and returning to your full awareness once more you can in your minds eye begin to sit up in your feather bed and stretch your arms above your head, stretch tall and long, that wonderful state that comes from stretching. Now swing your legs over the side of the bed and plant your feet firmly back on the ground.

It is time to climb back up those five steps, back to full awareness, back to your day. Standing up reading to go, it is time to climb, and when you reach the top in your minds eye, your physical body will be ready to leave this meditation journey and return to its normal functions.

Step up one step feeling more awake now, step up two, you are feeling really peaceful and confident that you can now control your sleep patterns and you know how to get the chaotic mind fall quiet, step up three, you have enjoyed your journey and your me time and are ready to face the day once more.

Step up 4 your body is feeling refreshed and awakened ready to take action. Step up five. You are full awake and have left your meditative state, you have taken a journey and learnt how to be the master of your sleep. Congratulations, now remember to practice your toy box technique daily!

Sleep 2

In order to get the maximum benefit from your meditation you first need to create a completely relaxed state and clear your mind of the hustle and bustle of daily life. Once you have found your comfortable place, close your eyes and focus on calming your breathing. Normal respiration is usually faster than we should breathe, however we rarely take time to focus on it.

Try and slow your breathing by focusing on the count of 4. Inhale for a count of 4.....1....2.....3....4......and exhale for a count of 4......1..... 2.....3......4.... Inhale for a count of 4.....1....2.....3....4......and exhale for a count of 4......1.....2.....3......4......every time you exhale try and release all tension and stress from your body, Inhale for a count of 4..... 1....2.....3....4......and exhale for a count of 4......1.....2.....3......4.... tensions escaping now, feeling calmer and more relaxed.

Just concentrate on your breathing, empty your mind of thoughts that can wait and instead listen to the meditation and use the power of your imagination to take you to wonderful places where stress doesn't exist and where you can develop your mind and being in the safety of a meditative state.

Now as you look around in your minds eye, you find yourself in a white room. A warm and inviting soft white sofa appears in front of you, and you stroll slowly over and sit down. Still taking in the sights around you.

On one wall is a beautiful ornate fireplace, with logs cracking and popping gently as they burn. The orange of the fire is the only colour in the room.

The room is deeply relaxing and peaceful.

Slowly a screen is lowered down in front of you, a large white television screen on a large white arm.

As screen flickers into life and you see before you a bedroom. This is not just any bedroom, this is your bedroom. The bed is perfectly made and it really does look warm and inviting. As you watch the screen the door of the bedroom swings open and you see yourself walk in. You look calm, calmer than you normally feel at bedtime, this is looking good. The you on the screen begins to get ready for bed.

Closing the curtains and switching to a less bright side light rather than the glare from the ceiling light. Your mobile phone has been left in the living area of your home, it is not a distraction that you need.

It decreases the chance of rest and increases the likelihood of sleep avoidance and you don't want that. You get ready for bed, pull back the duvet and sit in the bed. As you watch the you on screen begins to calmly repeat some positive affirmations. Tonight I will sleep soundly until I am fully rested. I trust the process of sleep. Sleep is good for every part of me. I enjoy sleep.

You are really enjoying seeing yourself looking this relaxed at bed time, you can see already that this version of you sleeps well. This version of you has a great relationship with rest and that makes you feel incredibly positive, you know that this is you, and therefore this is your future.

It is clear from the relaxed demeanour of the you on the screen that you easily and willingly release all the stresses of the day. You can see from your body language that you have a very relaxed manner and are clearly thinking about happy thoughts, this is how you have wanted sleep to be and you find it encouraging that this is what awaits you. You clearly have let go of all of your worries and really relish the chance to rest and sleep soundly at night.

The you on the screen is now laying in the bed looking perfectly at ease which is simply amazing - this is the sleep pattern and routine you have been craving and now you can see how to achieve it.

You can tell that the process of getting ready for bed and winding down is easy now. You are so relaxed as you finish your preparation for bed. You continue to watch the screen and to your surprise and delight the you on the screen falls asleep quickly and easily with no effort, no tossing and turning, no negative and stressful battles with yourself, just simply and easily sleeping as if it was the most natural thing in the world, which of course it really is.

You are just watching the you on the screen sleeping so peacefully, and you now feel peaceful and relaxed in yourself. This is how sleep should be and you know that this is something you can achieve after seeing this. The barriers to your own sleep seem to be fading away, and you now know that you will find this path to rest simply and easily. As you watch the screen the time on the clock speeds up and you notice that you are sleeping soundly as the hours tick by.

There is no waking or restlessness you just simply sleep naturally and soundly.

The clock ticks through the hours until morning arrives, and you watch as the you on screen awakens clearly relaxed and refreshed for having had such a brilliant sleep. You move nearer to the screen so wanting to be part of this scene you have been watching, you touch the screen and find you can pass through into the scene with ease.

As you become part of the scene you were just watching you feel suddenly calmer and more centred. You have an amazing positive state surge through you as you realise that this is you, and you have now worked out how to sleep peacefully and calmly, all night. You now know how to calmly prepare for bed and the positive way that you have seen know you can handle sleep. This reassures you that this is something you can now take forward and do for yourself.

You actually feel rested and revived yourself having watching the scene and now being part of it. Sleep has become a friend not an enemy and you release all negative emotions surrounding your bedtime routine. Sleep is now a positive time of day that you cannot wait to be part of. You know without doubt that you will be able to use this routine, absorb the calmness and serenity and you will now be able to head to be with such a positive knowledge of your ability to rest.

Increase Happiness

In order to achieve the best state of meditation let us first begin by relaxing the body and mind. Close your eyes and concentrate on the feeling of complete and total relaxation.

What does relaxation mean to you, today I want you to make relaxation the feeling of letting go, letting your muscles and body drain of tensions and stress. Working your way around your body think about how to let go and concentrate on letting each muscle and limb grow limp and lazy.

Your legs, your arms, fingers and toes, let them all grow limp, release all the tensions, let go of the stresses of the day, you do no need there here, there is no place for them in this here and now.

Right now, this is your time to relax and learn through the power of meditation. Today you are here to learn to focus on being happier, and that cannot happen if you bring with you all your worries and cares.

So for now, I want you to set aside any worries and cares, and as you concentrate on letting your body relax, I want you to allow your worries, your tensions, your stresses and your cares you drain from your body.

As they drain away you feel physically lighter, each and every muscle relaxes and lets go of stress and negativity and instantly feels lighter, draining the tensions is so good for the body, and you will notice how good it feels physically to be lighter and less bogged down by the tensions of the day.

You will notice how your breathing has become easier and deeper. This is a natural reaction to letting go of stresses and strains, your lungs relax and allow a more healthier breathing pattern to be established. As we go about our normal day our breathing is shallow and laboured - even if we are not concentrating on it, this is simply a reaction to the amount of things we try and pack into our lives.

Taking the time to focus on your breathing, especially at this time of mediation is really healthy for your lungs, see how relaxed your breathing has become, breathing as you do at night when you sleep soundly, peaceful and free.

Now I want you to see yourself in a room. This room has huge windows on three sides, and a couch along the back solid wall. The curious thing about this room is that everything is white. I want you to enter the room and cross to the white couch and sit down.

As you sit you notice your normal clothes have been replaced by flowing white robes. The room features a magical fireplace, standing freely in the centre of the room create the perfect amount of heat and light, even the coals are white. The only colour in the room comes from the orange of the flames as they dance. Settle yourself on the couch and look around.

Every window gives views of the most fantastic things, you will see a different view of scenes your truly love and enjoy out of each window. For some this is an amazing tropical beach, or a fantastic mountain view. Some people will see family playing and being happy. What you see will be what your heart truly loves, what makes you truly happy.

Enjoy these views for a moment. Feel at peace.

This room is the room of positivity. When you are in this room your thoughts can only be positive. This is the prefect space to focus on the positives of life and not the negatives. Seeing positives is a glass half empty technique - how you view a half filled glass is up to you.

If you choose to view the glass as half empty that is adopting an negative standpoint.

Equally you must learn to acknowledge that the glass is half full. Building a positive attitude to all situations will not only increase happiness but will make potentially difficult situations that bit easier.

This is the first technique you need to practice, and you can practice this every time you practice this meditation and you can practice this anytime of day but just bringing yourself to the room of positivity. The warmth and comfort, the white bright light of positivity.

You can begin to practice looking at any situation with positive eyes.

Imagine the dislike of winter, if you focus on this you can increase your stress and create a negative period for yourself where nothing seems right. However if you can focus on good things about winter you will create a better mental state. You can curl up in front of warm fires, you can wrap up warm and know you are returning to a lovely home later.

Simple changes to your thought processes can have a huge impact on how your view life.

Practise having gratitude for every blessing in life. Answer this question at least once a day, today I am grateful for......... It is down to you to fill in the blanks. Today I am grateful for loved ones, for friends, for the joy of simply being alive.

Try and find the answer to this statement at least once a day. As you count your blessings and express your gratitude enjoy being present and enjoying the moment. Look around your room of positivity and see all the positive and happy things through the windows. Enjoy being here, enjoy the moment.

Every time you come to this room you will find it easier and easier to explore the positive side of any situation. You will be able to learn how to let go of emotions and experiences which prevent happiness. You will be able to see how a thought, emotion or memory is actually empowering your negativity.

You will be able to use your new skills in positivity seeking to recognise a negative thought or emotion and over power it with positivity. There is no room here for negativity, this room does not allow negative thoughts. If you even begin to suspect a negative thought you need to immediately pop it into the fire and allow it to be destroyed.

Everything about this room is positive, you feel so positive being here. Whilst you are here I also want you to take time to focus on the positive in people rather than just in situations. See the best in yourself, identify what it is that makes you so amazing, because you are truly amazing.

Your love, your compassion, your gentle nature, your ability and desire to help others. This about what it is that makes you truly special. This is not your time to be modest, let yourself acknowledge your gifts and talents. You are not being proud or superior you are simply acknowledging to yourself what makes you the friend you are, the person you are.

Everyone of us is special and you are too.

This is perhaps the hardest exercise as people to do not like taking about themselves in such positive terms but it is important that you do so, and allow yourself to see how special you are. You can then do the same for your friends and family, and even strangers. Before you allow a negative thought to pop into your head look at the person and identity something positive about them.

This is especially important if someone has hurt you, the chances are it was accidental and instead of creating a cycle of negativity you need to restore positivity to balance

Seeing the best in yourself and others is another technique you may need to practice. You can practice this at anytime by using this room of positivity. You simply need to sit and enjoy the moment, sit and enjoy the room.

Look outside at the views that your inner self creates for you.

Enjoy watching these places that make you feel so good, enjoy watching the friends and family that make you feel so happy. Now enjoy creating positive thoughts and feelings about all the situations and people in your life. This maybe something you find an easy new skill or it might be something you have to work hard on. Sometimes we become convinced that a situation does not have anything positive about it but I want you now to challenge that.

Look again, look closely, for even the smallest spark of positivity is enough to light the flames of positive thought and bring about a whole new view point on a situation and increase your happiness. Finding your happy place, from the safety and comfort of this room of positivity will truly help you in all aspects of learning to be more positive. No matter how bleak you feel about a situation there is a positive element there somewhere. You just have to learn how to find it, grab hold of it, and build on it.

This is something that requires practice and you can return to this mediation at anytime to practice again, and enjoy being surrounding in positive thoughts and power. You can also summon yourself to this room in your mind at any time.

If you are living your daily life and a situation threatens to over power you with negative energy, you can transport you being to this place and practice the positive steps I have shown you. The more you practice the more confident you will feel. Focus your thoughts now back on the white room of positivity. Sit for the last few moments and completely immerse yourself in the wonderful atmosphere of such a positive place.

Enjoy the scenes playing outside the windows, your happy place. Enjoy them and notice how strong and peaceful you feel with this happy place held in your heart. It is time to leave this room now, but this room has become part of your mind and you can return here at any point in time. You can use the full meditation or your can train your brain to allow you to pop back when life threatens to overwhelm you.

It is time now to head to the door, walking now to the door, smiling at the experience of the room and enjoying the last glimpses of the wonderful scenes outside the windows, happy and peaceful in the knowledge you can come back at any time. Return your full awareness now back to the present moment, to your body, so relaxed and comfortable.

Remember these feelings, and how important it is to relax from time to time. Promise yourself, and mean it, that you will allow your body to return to this state often.

You owe it to yourself and it will help to keep you healthy and happy. The purpose is to increase happiness, and you have to love yourself and be kind to yourself in order to do this. You have to make time for your healing. Now you can focus on your physical body once more.

Slowly allow yourself to return to a full awareness as if you awakening from a deep and restful sleep. Begin to stretch your muscles and enjoy the state that follows complete relaxation. You are awakening now and will be able to return to the hustle and bustle of the day with a calmer more positive outlook and viewpoint.

You have done fantastic work today and you will benefit greatly from this. Congratulate yourself and enjoy the rest of your day.

Reduce Worry

Before we can begin the meditation we need to quiet the mind and create a state of relaxation. Close your eyes, and concentrate your thoughts on the here and now. Nothing else matters for the next half hour or so. Just you, being alone with yourself and yet pushing all thoughts and stress away as you sit quietly. There is no room here for stress and worry, you can leave those thoughts behind and instead focus on clearing your being, create an empty space with nothingness and light.

Once you have created a quiet mind it is time to take a journey, imagine a door in front of you, a pretty wooden door. Walk to the door and open it. Step thought the door and find yourself on an fantastic tropical island, a secret place only known to you here and now. You step out onto the sand, barefoot you can feel the soft warm sand beneath your feet. It is a glorious day, the sun is shining and the air is still, this really is an idyllic place to begin your meditative journey.

There is no one here to disturb you, the beach is calming and soothing, this really is a fantastic place to be and it is yours to use. Stroll lazily across the sand.

In the soft sand your feet sink a little, as you stroll down to the waters edge you notice the sand change to firmer moist sand and glancing behind you, you can see a trail of your footprints. The water feels warm on your feet as you wander lazily along the shore line just falling in love with this place. You are feeling so relaxed, this is a truly magical place that helps us learn and heal during meditation. There is nothing for you to worry about here, you have devoted this special time to yourself and that is truly valuable, you need to take time out to nurture yourself and develop yourself.

You are going to be learning valuable techniques to help you reduce worry. Before we begin just take a few more moments to enjoy the beach, stroll up and down the sand enjoying the contrast between the softest fine dry sand and the firmer moist sand by the shore line. You feel lazy and warm, its a very special place to be.

I want us now to think about worry. Not a specific worry, just the concept of worry. Firstly please be assured that everyone worries, it is a natural emotion that stems from our need to survive as prehistoric man. It is perfectly normal to worry but it is an emotion we need to control, and by using these techniques you will be better placed to control your worries and let go of the things you cannot control.

I want to show you a new way to view worry. I want you to stroll to a point on the beach where the sand is firm, but the water is close by. I want you to write your name in the sand. See your name in the sand, and now watch as the water laps higher, covering your name and washing it away.

This is how I want you to consider worry. The waves washing the beach were going to come no matter what action you took, so writing your name was actual quite futile. It was going to get washed away. We can use this trick to our advantage and help up consider things we worry about from a different point of view.

I want you to consider something simple. Imagine you have work on monday but you do not particularly like your job. If you spend your weekend worrying about work, in effect you are wasting your weekend and disallowing yourself happiness.

You understand the concept of time, so you know that after Saturday and Sunday comes Monday. There is nothing within your control you can do to change that. So stopping yourself enjoying your weekend only serves to harm you, your mental wellbeing, your stress levels etc.

If you choose to spend the weekend with friends and family enjoying the fact that these are not work days, you will arrive at Monday morning in a better mental place. So, on Friday night you can use your special beach, you can come here, walk in the sand and then when you are ready, write 'work' on the sand near the shore line.

Watch the water wash away the word work. As the word is washed away you must refocus your mind and not worry.

Until Monday morning work is not an issue that requires any of your attention. After all, until you actually get there you have no idea how the day will be. You might actually find you enjoy it! If you cannot control a situation you must learn to control the worry. If however a situation is within your influence then you can use more proactive methods to control the worry. Using our work analogy again, consider taking action to change your job. That is within your control.

By taking charge of the situation you can control your feelings of worry because you have taken steps to bring yourself away from that situation. Although several Mondays may have to come and go before you find another job, you know you are being active and handling problems that are within you influence.

So again on a Friday night you can return to your beach and release your worry about work and watch it wash away, but you can also go further up the beach where the water doesn't reach and start building your sandcastle of action that will take away the worry forever.

Practice now, in your safe place, writing your worries, worries that you know you cannot influence, writing them in the sand and watching the waves washing them away. Now consider the ways in which you could influence any worries, practical steps you can take on a situation you could influence. These practical steps are going to form turrets and building blocks on your sandcastle of action. Practice this for a while.

Visualise a worry, now ask yourself whether this is a situation that is within your control. If it is not something you can control or influence go down to the shore and write it in the sand, then stand back and watch the sea wash it away, and allow your feelings of worry to subside as it does so. This is nothing you can control therefore you should not be worrying, simply saving your energy for the outcome.

You cannot change the outcome, and in many cases you will not even really know what the outcome will be, therefore you need not concern yourself with it until it arrives. That is the time for action.

Do you remember a day in the past when you became consumed with a worry, a worry that you couldn't change, perhaps a fear of an exam, perhaps a dentist appointment. Looking back now do you see how insignificant this worry was. The day passed as all days do. You survived, you are here in the present. Did your worry change the outcome? In truth, if worry has any impact on situations we cannot control then sadly they will be only negative.

If we had phrased our exam nerves in terms of what we could do to influence the outcome, we would concentrate only on revision and technique to stay calm.. By using these techniques we may have influenced the situation in a positive way. However, if we became consumed with worry, we may have created a situation of negativity and under performed in the exam.

Remember the exam was a the situation we could not influence, it was going to happen regardless. How we handled that situation was within our control and influence so, had we gone down to the shore line, written exam, watched the sea wash it away, we would have done the best we possibly could to let go of that worry.

Had we then moved up the beach and revised, and built the sandcastle of action we would have cemented that positivity and presented at the exam in the best mental state possible.

But, even if you allowed worry to control that situation, now in the present it seems so insignificant and had so little impact can you see how worrying did not help in anyway? I think you can...so you can now build on this knowledge. There will still be situations that create a feeling of worry, but now you know how to best tackle these feelings.

Firstly ask yourself can I influence this situation - if you cannot then you need to write it in the sand and let it wash away - worrying changes nothing but your stress levels. If you can influence it then start building your sandcastle of action in the sand that cannot be reached by the water. You have control and are taking positive steps.

Finally remember to look back and think about situations you worried pointlessly over, as see how small and insignificant they have become with the passing of time. You are allowed to worry but you need to empower yourself to control that worry and use what you can change and wash away what you cannot change.

This is a powerful technique that you can summon at anytime, even if you do not have time, or are not in a suitable place to perform your full meditation you can simply in your minds eye see that warm beach, the section of sand on the shore line and write your worries there for them to be washed away. Allowing your worry levels to wash away at the same time.

Even in a crowded room, the more you can practice this visualisation, the more time you can return to this place of mediation the easier it will become for your to handle your worries quickly and efficiently sorting the things you can change from the things you cannot and acting accordingly. Seeing how a worry today will have faded into something so small and insignificant in just a short time in the future.

It is now time to leave this wonderfully place and return to your day. Remember though that you can recall this place at anytime, and you can commit to return to the full mediation regularly to help you address your worries. I want you now to wander back up the beach, back to the soft warm sand.

You can now see the doorway back to your room, back to your life. Open the door and step through. You have returned to your state of relaxation and empty thought.

You can now allow your body and mind to return to a full awareness once more, slowly and gently as if awakening from a deep restful slumber, stretching your body. Beginning with your toes and feet, ankles and legs, feel the wonderful sensation of stretching them out. Your hands and arm, your shoulders and neck, all the muscles stretching and relaxing. Stretch the muscles in your back, you are feeling wonderfully peaceful and relaxed and very positive about how you will tackle worry in the future.

You can now open your eyes and gently ease yourself back to reality - you have done great work and started a fantastic process - well done!

Winter log fire relaxation

The first thing we need to do is create a relaxed mind and body so that you can experience the deepest levels of relaxation possible. Begin by closing your eyes and focusing on your breathing. Concentrate on bring a peaceful and steady rhythm, breathing in 1, 2, 3 and breathing out 1, 2, 3. This can feel strange to start with as we are normally rushing around and never take the time to concentrate on our breathing.

Normal breathing is quite shallow, just enough to do the job. It is really good for our lungs to breathe a little deeper every now and then, and during a guided relaxation you have the perfect opportunity. With each breath that you take you can allow your muscles and body to relax a little bit more each time. Breathing in 1, 2, 3 and breathing out 1, 2, 3.

Allowing the cares of the day to slip away and your body to become more and more relaxed and rested. Keep concentrating on that breathing and enjoying the feeling of becoming more relaxed and more rested. Your body is relaxing and feeling nicely heavy and comfortable. You are ready to move on to deeper levels of relaxation.

Now in your minds eye I want you to imagine yourself in a wonderful forest on a snowy winter night. Although darkness has fallen the moon is full and bright and lights your way.

You can see clearly the trees and scenery around you. You are wrapped up warm in your winter coat and warm boots, but there is a better place you can be. Just ahead of you, you can see a small log cabin. There is smoke billowing gently from the chimney, the cabin is lit softly and it looks truly inviting. You instinctively know that this is your sanctuary and a wonderful place for you to go and spend sometime. You head towards the log cabin, your boots leaving deep prints in the snow behind you, your breath visible in the cool night air.

It is only a short stroll but you are still happy to reach the log cabin.

Pushing open the wooden door you are greeted by a wave of fabulously warm air. This really is the place to be. You step inside, and closing the door behind you, you pause to look around. An opulent but small space. On the back wall you can see the open fire that was creating the smoke you saw from outside. A heavy wooden mantle, with a deep crackling roaring fire below.

In front of the fire is a deep thick inviting fur rug, then a sofa cosy sofa with blankets and throws, and a fireside chair contain a blanket for your knees. All of them look so inviting. The rest of the cabin in quite simply laid out. A side table with a lamp, a door leading off here, a door leading off there.

They are of no interest to you at this moment, you are simply here to enjoy the warmth and comfort that a real fire brings. You can take off your big coat and snow boots and hang them by the door and sit wherever you feel drawn to sit.

Do you choose the sofa, the chair or perhaps the rug, to be as close as you can to this brilliant source of heat and light. Whatever you choose enjoy sinking into the soft seat of your choice. Glancing to the side you notice just beside you a mug of steaming hot chocolate. What a wonderful place this is.

You are already beginning to feel more relaxed than you were just a moment a go. The warmth uncurling all your limbs as you gently toast and warm your whole being Just sit for a moment and let your whole body absorb the warmth from the fire, you can really feel yourself getting warmer and feeling more relaxed even sleepy. Enjoy this state.

The fire gives the room a wonderful cosy glow, and the dancing flames are simply mesmeric. You stare into the fire and just watch how the flames dance and move. You can use these sights and sounds to find even deeper levels of relaxation. As you stare into the fire you can listen to the sounds a fire makes. Little pops and crackles as the logs burn.

All of these little pops and crackles are stresses and worries disappearing into the fire and spiralling up the chimney far far away from you. Imagine now any cares and worries, and places them like lumps of coal or small logs onto the fire. Do you see how easily they are taken and dealt with. No worry or care is to big or too difficult the fire pops and crackles and removes them all with ease. As each worry and care pops and crackles away you feel another bit of tension leave your body.

You feel a little heavier, but it is its a wonderful heavy state. You know this feeling means that you are learning how to relax deeper and deeper with every care that you let go here and now. This truly is a wonderful place, it is just for you. You can come back here anytime you want, and you should. You should vow now to make time to return to this amazing space regularly to allow your body and mind this deep relaxation that nourishes you and heals you. No one else is here to hassle you and you can enjoy being alone with the chance to relax and unwind.

You can just be you. Not a parent, not an employee, not a friend, not a child, none of life's roles need to come here with you. This is time for you just to be you and nothing else.

Do you feel how much more relaxed you are becoming as you let all cares and worries disappear onto the fire.

Notice how your muscles feel when you are this relaxed, notice how easy it is to breathe that slower and steadier rhythm. It all so much easier when you can relax, this should be your mantra and you should try to remember this when you are once more caught up in the hustle and bustle of life. It is some much easier when you can relax.

It is something we do not do enough so taking this opportunity is fantastic for your overall health and well being. No tension in the muscles means they feel wonderfully relaxed and lazy. The warmth of the fire helps you to relax even more. If any worries even so much as try and pop into your head simply toss them onto the fire.

Imagine them as logs or lumps of coal, and with a lazy movement throw them over onto the fire and watch as they pop and crackle and disappear into the cleansing flames. Watch as they become smoke and spiral up and up towards the chimney, up into the night sky and away from you forever.

You do not need them, you do not want them.

Let them go forever.

You can just enjoy sitting here feeling more relaxed than you can ever remember. Warm and cosy, nothing to do, no one calling you to action. This really is your time.

Time for you to nurture yourself and enjoy this amazing feeling of deep relaxation. You can take this state with you when you leave this place by remembering the popping and crackling of the fire, this will instantly leave you feeling calmer and more relaxed no matter where you are and what you are doing. relaxation is such a powerful trick to learn because the benefits to the body and mind are so healing and regenerating. It is so warm in front of the fire and you have become so relaxed that you are beginning to feel sleepy. You can fall asleep here all is safe and well.

When you awaken you have no idea how long you have been asleep but you become aware that you are back in your chair where you started this relaxation. You are waking up feeling so refreshed and so alive it is a wonderful state.

You can slowly begin to bring yourself back to full awareness once more. Stretch your limbs, enjoy the feeling the stretch creates. You are slowly waking up now and feeling so relaxed and peaceful. You can keep your eyes closed for a little longer and just enjoy feeling so warm and relaxed as you stretch your body.

See how long you can make your legs by stretching. See how high you can reach up as you stretch your arms.

Flex your neck form side to side, arch your back and allow your spine to stretch out. Doesn't that feel so good. Now you can allow your eyes to open and let your gaze gently scan the room as you adjust back to full awareness. What a wonderful skill you learnt today, well done!

Walking on a beach relaxation

First lets begin by closing your eyes. It is time to relax the body and prepare for the brilliant experience that lays ahead. Close your eyes and focus on your body. We need to release the stress that accumulates in daily life. Our muscles become tense and we hold ourselves stiffer and more upright the more that daily life stresses us. It is time to consciously release this stress. Time to allow the muscles to relax, come off guard.

All is well in this space and time. Here you need not worry about the problems of the day, you can simply leave them at the door. Here you need to simply allow yourself to relax. Give yourself permission to relax.

Relaxing is good. Feel the stress of the day draining from your body as you sink down into the chair or bed below you. Allowing the tensions to drain from the top of your head, much as you see sand run through an egg timer, allow the tensions to drain down, through the head and next, shoulders and back, arms and torso, thighs, legs and ankles, down through the floor, making you feel deliciously heavy and wonderfully relaxed and free of tensions.

Now I want you to come on a journey with me. A journey that will leave you more relaxed that you can ever imagine.

In your minds eye I want you to visualise the room you are in now. Imagine you are looking at the door, the door is closed. This is a magical door, the door to relaxation. This door has the power to take you to a wonderful place where you can experience total relaxation. All you have to do is follow the sound of my voice and allow the waves of relaxation to sweep over you.

In your minds eye I want you to see yourself walking towards the door. You believe you know where the doorway leads, this is your door, you have been through it many times, but today it has the power to transport you to amazing places. In your minds eye you are standing at the door with your hand on the handle. As you open the door you realise that you are no longer in your room, stepping out of your doorway. Instead you are walking through the doorway and finding yourself on a beach. Glancing behind you, you can see your room just as you know it.

It will still be there when you come back, but for now you are going to allow this magical doorway to transport you to this new place. Step through the doorway and notice the change of texture beneath your feet. You are stepping out into beautifully soft, warm sand.

You can close the door behind you, this is a wonderfully safe place.

You want to be here and experience the wonders of this new magical place. The beach seems to be part of a small island, you can see it curving away in front of you, and as you turn the other way it curves once more. You believe you could probably walk right around this island in the warm soft sand, and you would be right. This is your private island. It is not very big, but it is truly beautiful and filled with amazing natural beauty.

The temperature on the island is perfect for you. It is just as hot as you would choose a beach to be. As you step forward you notice you no longer have shoes or socks, and you can really enjoy the feelings of the soft warm sand on your toes. It is so peaceful here. There are no sounds of manmade distraction. No sounds of hustle and bustle.

All you can here are the waves gently lapping at the shore and the sound of birds calling as they soar and dive in the deepest of blue skies you can ever imagine seeing. The whole picture just adds to the sense of relaxation. There is nothing for you to do here except relax. No one to hassle you, no one to distract you. This is your time and your place to just experience relaxation.

Levels of relaxation that you didn't know existed. Levels of relaxation that we so often forget to allow ourselves to achieve.

For a moment I want you just to wander along the soft sand. Enjoy the feeling of the softest sand beneath your toes, enjoy the warmth and enjoy the solitude. It is so important to enjoy being alone occasionally. You are your best friend, you need to enjoy your own company. J ust enjoy slowly ambling through the sand looking at the sights around you. The sea as it laps the shore. The trees higher up the beach. The birds circling and singing. This is the most beautiful place you have ever seen. Such a perfect place to be.

Pick a place in the sand where you can just sit to watch the scenery. Notice how soft and supportive the soft sand is under your body weight. It cradles and supports you as you settle into a comfortable position. It is beautifully warm, and the rays of the sun provide your body with healing light. Vitamin D is vital for good health and you are here in the sun enjoying that light and warmth. Such a relaxing place.

Now I want you to reach down and take a handful of warm soft sand and let it trickle through your fingers. As you do this you can focus on letting your cares and worries become grains of sand. Let them slip away so easily and gently. Worries and cares are just barriers to achieving the fullest of relaxation, and you do not need them here and now, you can let them all go and remove the barriers to your own relaxation.

Picking up a handful of sand and watching it trickle through your fingers, repeating the process with a slow lazy deliberateness. You have no need to hurry, no need to worry, just time to relax and enjoy these feelings. Watching the sand trickling becomes mesmeric and soothing.

You can repeat this as many times as you like, moving sand from side to side, hand to hand. Allowing all of your tensions all of your stresses to fall away and be lost into the body of the beach, gone from your body, leaving you even more relaxed and feeling even more lazy. Remembering the sand trickling through your fingers is a great way to help you relax in day to day life.

Now I want you to pause for a moment and look at yourself. Look at how different you are when you are relaxed. There is no stress in your muscles, there is no tension in your shoulders or your stomach. There is a natural smile that occurs when you are this relaxed. It is an fantastic way to be and a state you can learn to find easily and simply using this guided relaxation.

Being totally relaxed brings so many benefits to the body and mind that it becomes an important skill. An important skill that is so enjoyable. Refocus yourself now back onto that beach, looking out into the distance and watching the waves lapping gently in and out, in and out.

So hypnotic you are becoming quite sleepy. You now feel more relaxed than you have ever been in your life. What a wonderful state. Free of worries and cares, ever muscle and fibre completely relaxed. You can now lay back into the sand and close your eyes. You can sleep and rest now you have cleared your mind and body of tension and stress. Relaxing more completely than ever before you feel so sleepy and so peaceful.

Your sleep rests you, and you start to regain awareness once more. You become aware that you are no longer on the beach but back in the safe and familiar surroundings of your room, sleeping and relaxing peacefully in your chair or bed. What an amazing adventure you have been on, and how many new skills you have learnt about relaxing the body completely. It is time now to return to full awareness once more.

You can take your time and do this nice and slowly. Like a blissful cat stretching out in front of the fire, uncurling all its limbs one by one, stretching them out. Eyes remain closed as you slowly start to uncurl and stretch. How wonderful a stretch is when you have been so relaxed. You feel so good.

Stretching out your arms and legs, twisting gently to release all of your muscles.

It really does feel good. You can now start to become aware of the sounds in the room, the familiar sounds you hear every day.

You can now open your eyes and slowly regain full awareness with your new found knowledge of relaxation.

You will find you can relax more easily and deeply every time you follow this meditation.

Enchanted forest relaxation

Before we can begin this wonderful journey to new levels of relaxation we first need to let go of the chaos of the day and quiet the mind from the chatter that happens endlessly in our minds. For now we need to be really strict and shut the chatter out. Close off the mind.

If it helps you imagine the 'Stop' signs you see in road repairs, imagine a big stop sign in your mind. Now turn that to face the chatter and the babble as that is not welcome for now. No thoughts or chatter can pass the stop signs, you create a void of space in your mind which is specifically and exclusively for now and for this moment of deep relaxation. There is no need to worry or give any time to the babble and chatter, it can wait and it will wait.

For now you need to just concentrate on being in the here and now. Allow your muscles to relax, allow your body to become heavy, and just allow the mind to remain empty and clear of all chatter. This is your time to experience great relaxation. Push aside all other thoughts they will wait.

Now I want you to imagine a door, a big wooden door, an intriguing door that makes you curious as to what lays behind it. In your minds eye go over to the doorway.

Push the door open and go and see what lays the other side. As you stroll through the door you find yourself in an enchanted forest. This is a beautiful magical place and you feel very lucky to be here. As you glance around you can see trees, bushes and many animals playing.

This is a very special enchanted forest and you are very lucky to be here. The trees have a lovely fresh piney scent about them. As you look ahead you can see a deer frolicking on the path ahead. Small brightly colour creatures seem to be flying from tree to tree collecting food.

You study them hard because you cannot be sure what they are.

Looking closer they seem to be some sort of fairy type creature. It is an enchanted forest so it really isn't any surprise that there are some weird and wonderful sights to be seen. You stop near a tree to watch the fairy folk at work. They are busy little creatures but seem quite happy that you are there. One of the flies gently round you head as if it is telling you something. It wants you to follow it further into the forest.

As you follow you find yourself feeling light and child like -there is no need for stress and worry in this place. Let yourself be free from stress and worry and skip off into the forest.

Still following the fairy you see lots of other creatures, mythical and enchanted creatures, it is as if you are in a fairy tale, what a beautiful way to spend time. You can see deer playing, rabbits hopping, it is so beautiful here. The sun is shining through the canopy of leaves over head. On one side you can see a stream babbling gently along the side of the forest.

Fish are jumping in and out of the crystal clear waters. The sound of flowing water is soothing and you feel even more relaxed as you enjoy your time in this amazing enchanted forest. Your fairy seems happy to wait for you as you take in all the sights and sounds, it really is quite unreal yet mesmeric here. There is something to see in every direction you look, all of nature looking perfect and beautiful.

Your walking pace has slowed as you are feeling so relaxed and easy now. Nothing to worry about here, no one needing you to just do them a quick favour. No one asking anything of you. This really is your time, just for you and no one else. Enjoy this time. Following the fairy you are taken to a clearing where there are blankets on the floor. It is so inviting you wander over and sit down. As you sit you realise that you have become even more relaxed that you all ready were. This is a lovely place that promotes relaxation, wellness and healing.

It is a great place to visit whenever you require a lift and to escape the daily grind of life. Looking up you see that leaves are gently falling from some of the trees, which is strange as it feels and looks like summer in the enchanted forest. Some of the leaves are red, some green, others shades of brown.

The falling leaves are so pretty as they spin and dance on their way down from the tops of the trees down to the forest floor. There are leaves falling and it dawns on you that these are worries and cares. We need to let our worries and cares fall away from us much like leaves fall from trees. Letting go and not thinking about them any more. You can practice this now.

Gaze up to the trees and concentrate your attention on a falling leaf, choose one, any one. As you choose a leaf transfer one of your worries or cares to the leaf and now watch it fall. Watch it fall all the way from the top of the tree down to the forest floor below. Watch as it lands amongst the other fallen leaves and is immediately lost amongst those already there. It becomes completely insignificant and invisible merged with all the other leaves on the forest floor. Now repeat this as many times as you require. Picking a leaf and watching it fall from the top of the tallest tree all the way down to the forest floor below. Blending with the others and becoming lost forever.

As you watch you cares and worries fall away see how much lighter you feel now you are not weighing yourself down with things that you cannot control. See how much better it is to simply let go and float the worries away. See how much more relaxed you feel. Your whole body becomes more and more relaxed. Your muscles, your fibres, even your cells feel so much more relaxed.

This is where healing occurs, this is where you can gain your strength and determination to hold on to this feeling of relaxation. To bring yourself back to this place again, often, anytime you need to watch worries and cares float away. Simply return to the enchanted forest where it is so easy, so very easy to let go of anything that troubles you. You sit for a while just watching the leaves fall from the top of the tallest tree to the bottom of the forest floor and disappear.

If any new worries or stressed creep past that stop sign you have put up in your mind then simply allocate them to a leaf and watch them disappear. You do not need to hang on to them, you do no want to hang on to them. You can safely let them go, and as you do so you awaken even deeper levels of relaxation that you did not even know you could achieve. This relaxation is so powerful and so good for your mind and your body you need to embrace it and treasure it now.

You just lay back watching the leaves falling, watching the pretty fairies playing and skipping overhead it is like being in a brilliant dream. Slowly you sit up, you decide that it is now time to leave this place and return to your day feeling so much more relaxed and prepared to handle anything that life chooses to throw at you.

You wander back along the path, and easily find the big wooden door that you now know leads to your room. Open the door and return to your original place. You can now start to return yourself to full awareness in order to continue your day. It is a bit like waking from a deep and restful sleep. There is no need to hurry, you have plenty of time and you can take as much time as you like to awaken yourself fully. You might want to start by gently stretching your arms and legs. It is an amazing feeling to relax fully and when you awake you may feel slightly tired but incredibly happy and contented.

Stretch out those limbs now and remember where you are, and what you are going to do next. Remember that this magical enchanted forest is there for you whenever you need to visit it.

The relaxation that we so often forget to allow ourselves it really very important to our over all health and well being.

As you stretch make a conscious decision to return to your place of

meditation every day, or as often as you possibly can. Enjoy relaxation!

Weight loss

Close your eyes and breath deeply. It is time to relax, time to release all the stress and strain of the day. As you relax concentrate on your breathing and notice how it begins to slow down. A peaceful state begins to envelope you like a big soft warm blanket. Clear your mind of all conscious thought.

Focus your attention on your room in your minds eye. Keeping your eye closed visualise the room around you that you know so well. The colours you have chosen, the pictures on the walls, you know without opening your eyes exactly where you have placed items of furniture.

As you visualise your room in your minds eye you become aware of a doorway that you haven't seen before. The doorway has a strangely welcoming feel about it, you just want to go over and see what is hidden behind, you just know it will be something good.

As you walk towards the door notice the colour, the door is your favourite colour, this makes you even more convinced that what lies behind it will be magical.

You feel a shiver of excitement as you reach for the door handle, what is behind this new door... you push the door open and stroll into a new room. You haven't seen this room before but it instantly makes you feel welcome and at ease, a lovely atmosphere. The unusual thing about this room is the fact the whole room is white.

No other colour at all, just a very peaceful but bright white. White walls, white floors, white ceilings, and a large white sofa. The room is surrounded on three sides with huge picture windows that look out onto wonderful scenes of tropical trees and beaches. The sun streams into the room, heating the room and making it feel even more inviting.

You stroll over to the large white sofa feeling drawn to sit, its is the most comfortable sofa you have ever sat on, you settle yourself down and notice a projector in front of you, its projecting onto the big blank wall, but at the moment there is no picture. Curious to see what the projector holds in store, you lean forward and press play.

The screen comes alive and the movie title flashes up. My ideal weight.

You realise that this movie is all about you!

As you watch in fascination you see yourself appear on the screen, the only difference between you now, and this you, is the weight. You are at your ideal weight and looking amazing!

As you continue to watch the screen, you watch yourself living your life, at a party, at work, going to the gym, what really strikes you is how you look - you are watching yourself with outsider eyes and you are so pleased with what you see. You are loving the way you look, the weight has gone, you look toned and fit.

The new weight loss seems to have given you a new found confidence too. You move with confidence, your head is held high, your shoulders are back, you look so great. As you watch yourself moving around at work and socialising you begin to notice that people are looking at you. You can tell they are looking at you positively. They are smiling as they interact with you, complimenting you on how fantastic you look. You cant help feel pride at your achievement, and the warm reaction you have been getting by friends and strangers alike.

The scene changes once more and you watch yourself at a large social event. On one side of this room is a large buffet table, overflowing with all sorts of foods.

You watch yourself approaching that table and wonder just what you are going to choose. You watch with surprise as your new slimmer self selects healthy salads, low fat meats and substantially less food than your know you eat at the moment. You watch as you carry the plate to a nearby table and sit with friends to eat. Again the new you surprises you further.

Food has been all consuming, you know you eat too much, too fast and food is a big focus in your life. This new you on the video seems different. Chatting and smiling your food has lost the focus you used to give it. When you do eat you slowly choose the right things, you take your time chewing them more, you seem relaxed and not obsessed with food. You adore watching these images, you thought losing weight would be impossible but this person on the screen seems to be finding it very simple. You notice that you haven't once glanced at the table for more food, that is unusual.

You are so total in awe of the situation you see before you that you stroll towards the screen, lifting your hand to touch the images in front of you. As you do you feel yourself being drawn into the seen floating above the room, watching yourself even closer. You are aware of how amazing you feel. Seeing yourself like this is filling you with so much motivation and determination.

You know that the only barriers to weight loss success is you, and you now know how you can remove those barriers and leave yourself free to see this vision become a reality. You now know that your daily mantra will be 'I see myself slim and healthy and therefore it will be' and that you now have the strength and determination to control your food and portion size better.

Floating above the room you now renew your commitment to a new healthier lighter you, you commit now to healthier eating knowing when you awaken and return to daily life you will find unhealthy food has lost its appeal. You want to be the you in the video and you now believe that it can and will happen. You are so excited to begin your new weight loss journey and you know without doubt you will succeed.

You turn and look back to the sofa and suddenly once more you are sat watching the screen, the time is now! You are keen to get back and begin. So, it is now time to leave this place and return to your daily life, filled with this new confidence and enthusiasm. It is time to start to bring your awareness back to the present moment. These images and experiences will never leave you they are engrained in your very being, etched on your memory.

They will be there to help you and motivate you, to keep you on track to success. With the images still very clear in your mind you can now return your focus to your breathing. See how incredibly relaxed your breathing has become whilst you have not been concentrating on it.

Bring your awareness back to your body and notice how relaxed your muscles are. Get contact with your hands and feet, gently move them, feel them awaking and stretching just as you do each morning when you awaken from a deep and restful sleep. Now continue the stretch to your legs and arms, your spine and neck, open your eyes and return to the room feeling successful and secure.

The Holistic Alchemist is happy to provide any of these meditations in a recorded MP3 format, with gentle backing music. Each track is £2.99

The Holistic Alchemist provides counselling, hypnotherapy, life couching and mediation services via Skype at £15 an hour.

To order any of the services please email anna@holisticalchemist.co.uk

Printed in Great Britain
by Amazon